The Role of Neuro-Linguistic Programming in Addressing Sleep Disorders

By Rex Morton

The Role of Neuro-Linguistic Programming in

Addressing Sleep Disorders

By Rex Morton

Disclaimer

This book is intended to provide information about the fields of Neuro-Linguistic Programming (NLP) and Cognitive Behavioural Therapy (CBT) and their potential integration. While the author has made every effort to ensure that the information was correct at the time of publication, the author does not assume and hereby disclaims any liability to any party for any loss, damage, or disruption caused by errors or omissions, whether such errors or omissions result from negligence, accident, or any other cause.

The contents of this book should not be used as a substitute for professional advice, diagnosis, or treatment. The reader should always consult with a qualified healthcare provider about any mental health concerns or conditions. Never disregard professional psychological or medical advice or delay in seeking it because of something you have read in this book.

The views expressed in this work are solely those of the author and do not necessarily reflect the views of the publisher, and the publisher hereby disclaims any responsibility for them.

The inclusion of websites, links, or references to other resources does not mean that the author or the publisher endorses the information the organization or website may provide or recommendations it might make. Furthermore, the author does not guarantee the accuracy of the information these resources provide.

The use of any information provided in this book is solely at your own risk.

A. Brief Overview of the Book

This book aims to explore the intriguing intersection of Neuro-Linguistic Programming (NLP) and sleep disorders. The chapters that follow will delve into the science of sleep, the concept of NLP, its potential impact on sleep disorders, and practical methods of using NLP techniques to improve sleep quality. By combining scientific research, real-life case studies, and practical strategies, we aim to provide a comprehensive understanding of how NLP can play a role in managing and treating sleep disorders.

B. Importance of Sleep for Health

Sleep is a fundamental requirement for the human body, impacting every aspect of our physical health and cognitive function. Quality sleep enables the body to restore and rejuvenate, to grow muscle, repair tissue, and synthesize hormones. In contrast, sleep deprivation or poor-quality sleep can lead to a host of health problems including heart disease, diabetes, obesity, depression, and impaired cognitive function. It's not just about the quantity of sleep; the quality, timing, and regularity of sleep also play critical roles in our wellbeing.

C. Explanation of Common Sleep Disorders

Sleep disorders are conditions that make it difficult for a person to get a good night's sleep, which can make them drowsy and dysfunctional during the day. Surprisingly, millions of individuals worldwide are affected by them. The most prevalent sleep disorders include insomnia (difficulty falling or staying asleep), sleep apnea (disrupted breathing during sleep), restless legs syndrome (an uncomfortable sensation leading to a need for constant movement of the legs), and narcolepsy (excessive, uncontrollable daytime sleepiness). These disorders can severely impact an individual's quality of life, leading to a wide range of health, mental, and emotional issues.

D. Introduction to Neuro-Linguistic Programming (NLP)

Neuro-Linguistic Programming, often referred to as NLP, is an approach to communication, personal development, and psychotherapy. It was created in the 1970s by Richard Bandler and John Grinder, who believed that there is a connection between neurological processes, language, and learned behavioral patterns. Through this approach, practitioners aim to 'reprogram' these learned behaviors to achieve specific goals in life. While NLP is sometimes seen as controversial, many individuals and therapists have found it to be a powerful tool for personal and professional development, and, as we will explore in this book, potentially a novel approach to addressing sleep disorders.

A. The Science of Sleep

Sleep is not merely a passive state of unconsciousness but a complex, dynamic process that affects every part of our lives.

i. Sleep Stages and Their Significance

Sleep can be divided into two main types: rapid eye movement (REM) sleep and non-rapid eye movement (NREM) sleep. Each type is linked to specific brain waves and neuronal activity.

There are three phases of NREM sleep. The transition from consciousness to sleep occurs during stage 1. Before transitioning to deeper sleep, stage 2 is a stage of light slumber. The third stage is profound slumber, and it is more difficult to awaken from this state. The body heals muscles and tissues, promotes growth and development, strengthens the immune system, and stores energy for the following day during this phase.

Following the NREM sleep stages, we move into REM sleep, often associated with vivid dreams. During REM sleep, the brain is active and dreaming occurs. This stage is essential for memory consolidation and mood regulation.

These sleep stages are cycled several times during the night, with each cycle lasting approximately 90-110 minutes.

ii. Circadian Rhythm and Its Role in Sleep

Our sleep-wake patterns are governed by an internal "clock" known as the circadian rhythm. This 24-hour cycle influences physical, mental, and behavioral changes, dictating not just our sleep patterns but also body temperature, hormone levels, and metabolism.

In a healthy state, our circadian rhythms coordinate with environmental cues like daylight and darkness to encourage predictable cycles of sleeping and alertness. Sleep difficulties can result from changes to this cycle, such as those brought on by shift work, jet lag, or certain illnesses.

B. Prevalence and Impact of Sleep Disorders

Sleep disorders, affecting a substantial portion of the global population, can have significant impacts on health and daily life.

i. Types of Sleep Disorders: Insomnia, Sleep Apnea, Restless Legs Syndrome, and more

Insomnia, characterized by difficulty falling asleep or staying asleep, is one of the most common sleep disorders. Sleep apnea, another prevalent disorder, involves interrupted breathing during sleep, resulting in reduced oxygen flow to the brain. The neurological condition known as restless legs syndrome (RLS) is characterized by a strong impulse to move the legs when inactive, frequently interrupting sleep. Extreme daily sleepiness and brief periods of sleepiness are symptoms of the severe but less common disorder narcolepsy.

ii. Effects of Sleep Disorders on Physical, Mental, and Emotional Health

Sleep disorders can cause a range of health problems. Physically, they can lead to an increased risk of cardiovascular disease, obesity, and weakened immune function. Mentally, sleep disorders can contribute to issues such as depression, anxiety, and cognitive impairment. Emotional impacts can include mood swings, decreased motivation, and increased irritability.

iii. Societal and Economic Impacts of Sleep Disorders

The societal impacts of sleep disorders are far-reaching. Beyond the direct health consequences, these disorders can lead to decreased productivity, increased accident risk, and strained interpersonal relationships. The economic costs are also considerable, with billions spent each year on direct medical costs related to sleep disorders, not to mention the indirect costs due to lost productivity and accidents.

Understanding the nature and impact of sleep and sleep disorders is the first step toward identifying potential treatment strategies, such as Neuro-Linguistic Programming, which will be discussed in the following chapters.

A. History of NLP

Neuro-Linguistic Programming (NLP) was conceived in the 1970s by Richard Bandler, a psychology student, and John Grinder, an assistant professor of linguistics. Their goal was to model and decode the thought processes and behaviors of effective and successful individuals, believing that these could be learned and replicated by others.

They began by observing psychotherapists, particularly Virginia Satir, Fritz Perls, and Milton Erickson, who had a reputation for obtaining outstanding results. Through rigorous analysis of their methods, Bandler and Grinder developed a series of tools and techniques which they coined as Neuro-Linguistic Programming, representing the interaction between the mind (neuro), language (linguistic), and behavior (programming).

B. Principles and Techniques of NLP

NLP comprises various principles and techniques, each designed to understand and alter patterns of thought, behavior, and communication.

i. Sensory Acuity and Calibration

Sensory acuity in NLP refers to a practitioner's ability to notice, observe, and interpret the non-verbal responses of others, such as changes in skin color, body language, or tone of voice. Calibration, on the other hand, is the process of associating these observable behaviors with an individual's internal states. Together, they enable a practitioner to understand the emotions and thoughts of others beyond explicit verbal communication.

ii. Rapport, Pacing, and Leading

Rapport is the feeling of trust and understanding in a relationship. In NLP, practitioners establish rapport with clients by matching or mirroring their behaviors, language, or beliefs. Once rapport is established, practitioners can use 'pacing' to match the client's current state and 'leading' to guide them towards desired changes.

iii. Representational Systems

NLP recognizes that individuals represent their experiences through sensory perceptions, primarily visual, auditory, kinesthetic, olfactory, and gustatory. Understanding a person's primary representational system (the preferred way to process information) allows practitioners to communicate more effectively and facilitate change.

iv. Anchoring, Reframing, and Future Pacing

Anchoring in NLP involves creating a stimulus-response association. For example, a certain gesture or word can be used to trigger a particular emotional state. Reframing involves changing the context or meaning of an experience to alter its emotional impact. Future pacing, on the other hand, is a method where the client mentally rehearses desired behaviors and outcomes to increase the likelihood of their actual occurrence.

C. The Role of NLP in Therapy and Personal Development

NLP is often employed as a therapeutic tool. It is used to help individuals understand their thinking and behavioral patterns, and to develop strategies for positive change. By learning to use language and thought more effectively, individuals can overcome limiting beliefs, phobias, or behaviors. Moreover, NLP techniques like reframing and anchoring can be used to instill new, more productive habits.

In personal development, NLP can help individuals improve communication skills, build rapport, set and achieve goals, and increase self-awareness. It can be particularly useful in fields such as leadership, sales, coaching, and sports psychology.

D. Controversies and Criticisms of NLP

Despite its widespread use, NLP has been subject to criticism and controversy. Some researchers question its scientific validity, citing a lack of rigorous empirical evidence supporting its effectiveness. Critics also argue that NLP is overly simplistic, reducing complex human behaviors and experiences to mere patterns and strategies.

Furthermore, the field of NLP has been criticized for lack of standardization in training and certification, leading to variance in the quality of NLP practitioners.

However, despite these criticisms, many practitioners and clients attest to the positive impacts of NLP, and it continues to be a popular tool in therapy and personal development. The potential applications of NLP, including its use in managing sleep disorders, remains an area of interest for practitioners and researchers alike.

A. Role of the Mind in Sleep Patterns

The mind plays a significant role in the regulation of sleep patterns. Mental states and thought processes can either promote restful sleep or contribute to sleep disturbances. Stress, worry, and anxiety are commonly associated with insomnia and other sleep disorders. These negative emotional states can elevate arousal levels, making it harder to fall asleep or maintain uninterrupted sleep.

On the other hand, relaxation, calmness, and positive mental imagery can facilitate the transition into sleep and promote a more restful sleep experience. Hence, understanding and harnessing the power of the mind becomes an important tool in managing sleep disorders.

B. Use of NLP in Modifying Sleep-related Behaviors

NLP provides a toolkit of techniques that can be used to influence sleep-related behaviors. For example, NLP's reframing techniques can help people change their perceptions of bedtime, shifting it from a source of stress and anxiety to a welcome opportunity for rest and rejuvenation.

Anchoring can also be used to create positive associations with sleep. For instance, a particular relaxation routine or calming mental image could be 'anchored' to the state of feeling sleepy, allowing individuals to trigger this state at will.

Sensory acuity and calibration can help individuals become more aware of their own physiological and mental states that precede sleep, enabling them to facilitate these states. Additionally, by understanding an individual's representational systems, NLP practitioners can provide personalized techniques for inducing sleep, such as guided visualizations for those who are visually oriented or calming auditory suggestions for those who respond well to sound.

C. Hypothetical Case Studies Showing NLP's Application in Sleep Improvement

Case Study 1: Insomnia

John, a 35-year-old software engineer, suffered from chronic insomnia. He associated bedtime with stress and often lay awake for hours with racing thoughts. An NLP practitioner worked with John to reframe his negative associations with sleep. They used anchoring techniques to link a pre-sleep routine - a warm bath and calming music - to feelings of relaxation and sleepiness. Over time, John reported a significant improvement in his sleep quality and a decrease in bedtime anxiety.

Case Study 2: Sleep Apnea

Sarah, a 45-year-old woman, had sleep apnea and often woke up feeling tired and groggy. After unsuccessful attempts with traditional treatments, she sought help from an NLP practitioner. The practitioner taught Sarah relaxation techniques and calming visualizations (based on her primary representational system) to help her fall asleep more easily after the interruptions caused by her sleep apnea. They also worked on reframing her negative feelings about her disorder, which had been causing her additional stress. Although NLP couldn't cure the sleep apnea, Sarah reported that she felt better rested and less anxious about her sleep disorder.

These cases illustrate how NLP techniques can be tailored to individual needs and circumstances to address sleep disorders. While further research is needed, NLP offers promising tools for improving sleep by harnessing the power of the mind.

A. Identifying and Setting Sleep Goals with NLP

The first step in using NLP for sleep disorders is identifying and setting clear, achievable sleep goals. For instance, a person with insomnia may set a goal to fall asleep within 30 minutes of getting into bed, while a person with sleep apnea might aim to feel more refreshed upon waking.

NLP goal setting is often based on the SMART principle, meaning goals should be Specific, Measurable, Achievable, Relevant, and Time-bound. For example, instead of setting a goal like "I want to sleep better", a SMART goal would be "I will sleep for at least 7 hours per night for the next month".

B. NLP Techniques for Dealing with Insomnia

For dealing with insomnia, the NLP technique of reframing can be useful. Reframing involves changing one's perception of a situation to alter its emotional impact. For instance, if a person dreads bedtime due to the anticipated struggle with sleep, they could reframe it as a time to rest and relax, regardless of whether sleep comes immediately.

Anchoring, another NLP technique, can also be used to promote sleep. An individual might anchor a state of relaxation to a specific bedtime ritual, like reading a book or listening to calming music. Over time, the ritual triggers the relaxation response, helping the person fall asleep more easily.

C. NLP Techniques for Dealing with Sleep Apnea

While NLP can't cure sleep apnea, it can help manage the stress and frustration associated with this disorder. Techniques such as rapport building and future pacing can be beneficial here. The NLP practitioner would build a trusting relationship with the client (rapport), then guide them through a visualization process where they see themselves managing the condition effectively in the future (future pacing).

Another useful NLP tool could be the use of metaphor or story-telling. This can create new patterns of thought and enable the client to see their situation from a different perspective, often leading to a reduction in stress and anxiety associated with their condition.

D. NLP Techniques for Dealing with Other Sleep Disorders

In the case of Restless Leg Syndrome (RLS), NLP can be used to help individuals manage the uncomfortable sensations that disturb their sleep. Visualization techniques can be used to distract the mind from the uncomfortable sensations, or even to reimagine them in a less distressing way.

For Narcolepsy, where individuals experience excessive daytime sleepiness, techniques like future pacing can be helpful. This technique can help individuals visualize themselves staying awake and alert during the day, which can then influence their actual ability to do so.

In all cases, it's important to note that while NLP can provide useful tools for managing and coping with sleep disorders, it should not be considered a replacement for medical advice or treatment. Always consult a healthcare provider for a comprehensive treatment approach to sleep disorders.

A. Case Study 1: Overcoming Insomnia with NLP

Mary, a 40-year-old teacher, has been struggling with chronic insomnia for several years. Her sleep is plagued by persistent worries about work, which causes her to lay awake for hours every night. Her NLP practitioner begins by setting sleep goals with her, aiming to help Mary fall asleep within 30 minutes of going to bed. They use reframing techniques to help Mary see bedtime as a relaxation period rather than a time for worrying about work. Anchoring techniques are also applied, associating the act of reading a calming book with the onset of sleep. After several weeks of applying these techniques, Mary reports significant improvement in her sleep onset time and overall sleep quality.

B. Case Study 2: Managing Sleep Apnea with NLP

David, a 55-year-old accountant, suffers from obstructive sleep apnea. He feels frustrated and anxious about his interrupted sleep, leading to further sleep disturbances. His NLP practitioner uses rapport building to develop a trusting relationship, then applies future pacing. David is guided to visualize himself managing his sleep apnea effectively, waking up refreshed and invigorated. They also use storytelling to help David change his perspective on his condition, reducing associated anxiety. After a few months of NLP therapy, David reports a decrease in his stress levels and improved overall sleep quality, despite the continued presence of sleep apnea.

C. Case Study 3: Tackling Restless Legs Syndrome with NLP

Laura, a 30-year-old software developer, has Restless Legs Syndrome that disrupts her sleep nightly. Her NLP practitioner uses visualization techniques to help Laura manage the uncomfortable sensations that keep her awake. Laura is guided to imagine the sensations as energy waves that she rides smoothly, transforming a distressing experience into a manageable one. This change in perception, along with improved sleep hygiene practices, results in Laura experiencing fewer sleep disruptions and improved overall sleep.

D. Evaluating the Success and Limitations of NLP in these Case Studies

In these case studies, NLP techniques played a significant role in improving the sleep quality of individuals struggling with different sleep disorders. Through reframing, anchoring, future pacing, and visualization, the individuals were able to alter their perceptions, manage their symptoms more effectively, and improve their sleep.

However, it's important to recognize the limitations of these cases. NLP was used as a complementary tool in conjunction with other sleep hygiene practices and, where necessary, medical treatment. While NLP techniques can help manage the symptoms and psychological aspects of sleep disorders, they are not a cure for the physical causes behind some sleep disorders, such as sleep apnea or Restless Legs Syndrome. Furthermore, the effectiveness of NLP can vary from person to person, depending on factors such as their openness to the techniques and their relationship with the NLP practitioner.

These cases highlight the potential of NLP as part of a holistic approach to managing sleep disorders, offering valuable strategies for those who find traditional treatment methods insufficient.

A. Conventional Treatments for Sleep Disorders: Medications, Sleep Hygiene, and Cognitive Behavioral Therapy

Conventional treatments for sleep disorders typically involve a combination of medication, sleep hygiene, and cognitive behavioral therapy (CBT).

Although they can offer temporary relief, medications like sleeping tablets don't address the underlying cause of sleep issues and can have negative effects. In order to sleep well, one should practice good sleep hygiene, which includes following a regular sleep schedule, abstaining from coffee in the hours before bed, and establishing a sleep-friendly environment.

CBT for insomnia (CBT-I) is considered the gold standard treatment for chronic insomnia. It involves techniques like sleep restriction, stimulus control, and cognitive restructuring to break the cycle of sleeplessness.

B. Alternative Treatments: Acupuncture, Hypnosis, and Yoga

Numerous alternative therapies, including yoga, hypnosis, and acupuncture, provide various strategies for enhancing sleep. Acupuncture is a form of traditional Chinese medicine that includes inserting needles into the body at particular locations in an effort to promote healing and restore balance.

Hypnosis, often confused with NLP, involves inducing a state of deep relaxation and using suggestions to influence behavior, thoughts, or perceptions. While similar, NLP is broader, incorporating elements of hypnosis but also drawing from other disciplines.

Yoga promotes better sleep by combining physical postures, breath control, and meditation to reduce stress and promote relaxation.

C. NLP versus Conventional and Alternative Treatments: Strengths, Weaknesses, and Suitability

Comparatively, NLP provides a unique approach to managing sleep disorders by focusing on changing thought patterns and behaviors. Like CBT, it involves cognitive restructuring, but NLP is more flexible, allowing techniques to be customized to an individual's specific needs and preferences.

NLP has strengths and weaknesses compared to other treatments. Its main strength lies in its ability to provide personalized strategies for managing sleep disorders. It can be particularly useful for those whose sleep issues are closely tied to stress, anxiety, or negative associations with sleep.

However, a key weakness of NLP is the lack of robust scientific evidence supporting its effectiveness. While many people find it helpful, the results can vary widely. Furthermore, it does not treat the physiological aspects of some sleep disorders, like sleep apnea.

Conventional and alternative treatments each have their place. For instance, medication may be necessary in acute cases, while sleep hygiene should form the foundation of any sleep improvement strategy. CBT-I has strong evidence supporting its effectiveness for insomnia. Alternative treatments like acupuncture, hypnosis, and yoga can be helpful for some individuals, although the scientific evidence varies.

The suitability of NLP or any other treatment modality depends on individual factors, including the nature and severity of the sleep disorder, the person's preferences, their responsiveness to different treatments, and their overall health condition. As always, any treatment for sleep disorders should be undertaken in consultation with a qualified healthcare provider.

A. Advancements in NLP Techniques

As our understanding of the human mind expands, so too do the techniques available within the NLP framework. Future advancements in NLP may involve the integration of emerging technologies. For instance, virtual reality could potentially be used to create immersive experiences that enhance NLP exercises, such as visualization and future pacing.

In addition, ongoing refinements in existing NLP techniques will continue to emerge from the shared experiences of practitioners. For instance, NLP anchoring techniques might evolve to become more effective and nuanced, or new ways of reframing sleep-related thoughts may be discovered.

B. Current Research and Potential Developments in NLP for Sleep Disorders

While NLP is not traditionally a research-driven field, there is an increasing interest in scientifically investigating its effects. Current research efforts are looking at the measurable impact of NLP techniques on various aspects of health and well-being, including sleep.

Future research could provide more insight into the mechanisms through which NLP impacts sleep and uncover new applications for NLP in the management of sleep disorders. This might involve rigorous clinical trials comparing NLP to other treatments, or studies exploring the long-term effects of NLP on sleep quality.

C. Integrating NLP with Other Treatments

Perhaps the most promising direction for the future of NLP in sleep disorder management is its integration with other treatment modalities. For instance, combining NLP with CBT-I could offer a more holistic approach, addressing both cognitive and behavioral aspects of insomnia.

Similarly, integrating NLP with sleep hygiene education could help individuals to not only learn about good sleep habits but also address any subconscious barriers to implementing these habits. In cases of sleep disorders linked to physical conditions, such as sleep apnea, NLP could be used alongside medical treatment to help manage associated stress and anxiety.

Furthermore, advances in telemedicine and digital health platforms could make NLP more accessible to a wider audience. This could involve online NLP sessions, apps that guide individuals through NLP exercises, or digital support groups for people using NLP to manage their sleep disorders.

As we continue to explore the complexities of sleep and its disorders, it's clear that NLP offers a unique and valuable toolkit. Its future in sleep disorder management looks promising, and ongoing advancements and research are likely to further refine its role in this field.

A. Summary of Key Points

This book aimed to explore the role of Neuro-Linguistic Programming (NLP) in addressing sleep disorders. We began by understanding the science of sleep and the impact of sleep disorders on individuals and society. We then dove deep into the concept of NLP, its principles, techniques, and its role in therapy and personal development. The subsequent chapters focused on how NLP intersects with sleep, how its techniques can be applied to manage various sleep disorders, and shared hypothetical case studies demonstrating its potential efficacy.

We further compared NLP with other conventional and alternative treatment modalities, highlighting its unique strengths and weaknesses. Finally, we discussed the future of NLP in managing sleep disorders, emphasizing the importance of advancements, current research, and integration with other treatments.

B. The Potential of NLP in Addressing Sleep Disorders

NLP offers a unique approach to managing sleep disorders, focusing on changing thought patterns and behaviors that contribute to these conditions. Through its flexible and customizable nature, NLP has the potential to address the individual-specific psychological aspects of sleep disorders. However, like any other treatment modality, it's not a one-size-fits-all solution and should be considered as part of a broader, holistic approach to sleep disorder management.

C. Final Thoughts and Encouragement for Continued Research and Application

While NLP shows promise in the realm of sleep disorder management, there's still much to explore. It's our hope that this exploration encourages continued research into NLP's effectiveness, mechanisms, and best practices, leading to better, more evidence-based applications of this tool in sleep disorder treatment.

Moreover, it's important for clinicians and individuals alike to remain open to a variety of treatment modalities. Sleep disorders are complex conditions that often require a multifaceted approach. NLP, in conjunction with other treatments, may offer new hope for those struggling with these challenging conditions.

In the end, the journey to better sleep is a personal one, and NLP could be an empowering part of that journey for many. So, let's continue to learn, grow, and explore the possibilities this unique tool has to offer in our quest for restful and restorative sleep.

Rex Morton is a renowned author and researcher in the United Kingdom with a passionate interest in the human mind, specifically in Cognitive Behavioural Therapy (CBT) and Neuro-Linguistic Programming (NLP).

Morton has spent a considerable portion of his professional life diving deep into the theories and principles that form the backbone of these two compelling fields. His fascination with NLP led him to complete an extensive certification program, solidifying his understanding of this innovative approach to understanding human behaviour.

Although Morton does not have clinical experience, his intense curiosity and dedication to studying these subjects have made him a respected figure in the field. He has thoroughly researched the integration of NLP techniques into CBT, offering fresh perspectives and insights into how these two methodologies can complement each other to enhance understanding of human cognition and behaviour.

As an author, Morton has successfully communicated his knowledge and passion to a broader audience, making complex psychological theories accessible to professionals and interested laypersons. His writing is characterized by a clear, engaging style and a focus on the practical application of theories, making them relevant to everyday life.

In his personal life, Morton is an ardent lover of the natural world, often spending his free time exploring the British countryside. His passion for landscape photography allows him to capture and share the beauty of these excursions. Despite his accomplishments, Morton is known for his humility and eagerness to continue learning. His work continues to inspire those interested in the intricate workings of the human mind and the exciting possibilities presented by the integration of NLP and CBT.

If you've found the content of this book enlightening and wish to continue your journey of understanding the human mind, I warmly invite you to visit my website at www.rexmorton.com. The website serves as a hub of knowledge where I share my latest findings, thoughts, and insights on the integration of NLP and CBT.

I also encourage you to subscribe to the newsletter available on the website. By subscribing, you'll receive regular updates on a range of topics, from detailed discussions on specific NLP techniques and their application in CBT, to the latest research in the field.

The newsletter is also the first place I'll share news of upcoming releases. Whether it's the announcement of a new book, the launch of an online course, newsletter subscribers will be the first to know. This is a great opportunity to continue learning directly from me, deepening your understanding of NLP and CBT, and enhancing your skills in applying these techniques in your own life or professional practice.

I'm looking forward to sharing this journey with you.

9 798863 369068